HPLC Basics

www.lulu.com
Lulu Press, Inc
627 Davis Drive, Suite 300,
Morrisville, NC 27560.

Author Affiliations

Mr. Upender Rao Eslawath,
Associate Professor,
Department of Pharmaceutical Analysis,
Vikas College of Pharmacy,
Jangaon, Telangana, India-506167.

Dr. Rajashekar Vadlakonda,
Associate Professor,
Department of Pharmaceutical Chemistry,
Vikas College of Pharmacy,
Jangaon, Telangana, India-506167.

Mr. Saarangi Ramesh
Associate Professor
Department of Pharmaceutical Chemistry,
Vijay College of Pharmacy,
Nizamabad, Telangana, India-503003.

First Printing: 2023
ISBN: 9781312463653
Copyright License @ Upender Rao Eslwath

This book has been published with all reasonable efforts to make the material error-free after the author's consent. No part of this book shall be used or reproduced in any manner, without the author's permission, except for brief quotations embodied in critical articles and reviews.

The Author of this book is solely responsible and liable for its content, including but not limited to the views, representations, descriptions, statements, information, opinions, and references ["Content"]. The Content of this book shall not constitute or be construed or deemed to reflect the opinion or expression of the Publisher or Editor. Neither the Publisher nor Editor endorse or approve the Content of this book or guarantee the reliability, accuracy, or completeness of the Content published herein and do not make any representations or warranties of any kind, express or implied, including but not limited to the implied warranties of merchantability, fitness for a particular purpose. The Publisher and Editor shall not be liable whatsoever for any errors or omissions, whether such errors or omissions result from negligence, accident, or any other cause or claims for loss or damages of any kind, including without limitation, indirect or consequential loss or damage arising out of use, inability to use, or about the reliability, accuracy or sufficiency of the information contained in this book. This book was written based on intelligence with the support of various sources.

HPLC Basics

By

Mr. Upender Rao Eslawath

Dr. Rajashekar Vadlakonda

Mr. Saarangi Ramesh

Lulu
2023

About the Author

Mr. Upender Rao Eslawath is an Associate Professor with 13 years of teaching experience. He authored 13 papers in international and national Journals. He has two international Patents. He presented and participated in various national and international conferences. He has five years of research experience and guided 9 PG students. He is expertise in handling various analytical instruments like HPLC and UPLC.

Dr. Rajashekar Vadlakonda is an Associate Professor with 14 years of teaching experience. He authored 16 papers in national and international journals. He has three international patents. He also presented and participated in many various national and international conferences. The Universities appointed him as an adjudicator at various National conferences. He has eight years of research experience and guided 12 PG students and two research scholars.

Mr. Saarangi Ramesh is an Associate Professor with thirteen years of teaching experience. He authored 17 papers in national and international journals. He has one international patent. He has seven years of research experience and guided 6 PG students. He also presented and participated in various national and international conferences.

About Book

This book describes the powerful analytical technique, i.e., HPLC, used to separate, identify, and quantify components in a mixture. This book is helpful for various fields, including pharmaceuticals, biochemistry, environmental analysis, food and beverage testing, and forensics. This book discusses the types of HPLC apparatus, their use, components, standard operating procedures, and their limitations.

Table of Contents

High-Performance Liquid Chromatography 1
    Introduction 1
    Types of HPLC 3
A. Reverse-Phase Chromatography 6
    Introduction 6
    Components of Reverse-Phase Chromatography 7
    Standard Operating Procedure of Reverse-Phase Chromatography 9
    Limitations of Reverse-Phase Chromatography 11
B. Normal-Phase Chromatography 14
    Introduction 14
    Components of Normal Phase Chromatography 16
    Standard Operating Procedure of Normal Phase Chromatography 17
    Limitations of Normal Phase Chromatography 20
C. Ion-Exchange Chromatography 22
    Introduction 22
    Components of Ion-exchange Chromatography 24
    Standard Operating Procedure for Ion Exchange Chromatography 25
    Limitations of Ion-exchange Chromatography 28
D. Size-Exclusion Chromatography 30
    Introduction 30
    Components of Size-Exclusion Chromatography 31
    Standard Operating Procedure of Size-Exclusion Chromatography 33
    Limitations of Size-Exclusion Chromatography 35
E. Chiral Chromatography 37

    Introduction 37

    Components of Chiral Chromatography 38

    Standard Operating Procedure of Chiral Chromatography 40

    Limitations of Chiral Chromatography 42

F. Affinity Chromatography 45

    Introduction 45

    Components of Affinity Chromatography 46

    Standard Operating Procedure of Affinity Chromatography 48

    Limitations of Affinity Chromatography 51

G. Hydrophilic Interaction Chromatography 53

    Introduction 53

    Components of Hydrophilic Interaction Chromatography 54

    Standard Operating Procedure of Hydrophilic Interaction
    Chromatography 55

    Limitations of Hydrophilic Interaction Chromatography 58

H. Hydrophobic Interaction Chromatography 61

    Introduction 61

    Components of Hydrophobic Interaction Chromatography 62

    Standard Operating Procedure of Hydrophobic Interaction
    Chromatography 64

    Limitations of Hydrophobic Interaction Chromatography 66

I. Multimodal Chromatography 68

    Introduction 68

    Components of Multimodal Chromatography 70

    Standard Operating Procedure of Multimodal Chromatography 71

    Limitations of Multimodal Chromatography 74

HPLC Basics

HPLC Basics

High-Performance Liquid Chromatography

Introduction

High-Performance Liquid Chromatography (HPLC) is a powerful analytical technique used to separate, identify, and quantify components in a mixture. It is widely employed in various industries, including pharmaceuticals, chemistry, food and beverage, environmental analysis, and forensic science.

HPLC is based on the principles of liquid chromatography, where a sample mixture is dissolved in a solvent and injected into a column packed with a stationary phase. The column contains small particles coated with a stationary phase material, which interacts differently with the components of the sample mixture. As the mobile phase (solvent) is pumped through the column at high pressure, the sample components are separated based on their differential interactions with the stationary phase.

Key Components of an HPLC System

Mobile Phase: The solvent or a mixture of solvents carries the sample through the system. Selecting an appropriate mobile phase is crucial for achieving desired separation and elution of analytes.

Stationary Phase: The stationary phase is a material coated on the surface of the particles within the column. It interacts with the sample components based on their chemical properties, such as polarity, charge, or size.

Column: The column contains the stationary phase and provides a separation platform. It is typically a stainless-steel tube packed with small particles, usually a few micrometers in size, to maximize the surface area for interactions between the sample and stationary phase.

Pump: The pump delivers the mobile phase at a constant flow rate, typically at pressures ranging from 1000 to 5000 psi, ensuring a consistent elution of the sample components through the column.

Injector: The injector is responsible for manually introducing the sample into the mobile phase flow or through an autosampler, which allows for automated and precise sample injections.

Detector: The detector detects and quantifies the separated sample components as they elute from the column. Depending on the analyte's nature and detection requirements, various detectors are used in HPLC, including UV-Visible, fluorescence, refractive index, and mass spectrometers.

Data System: The data system or chromatography software controls the instrument, processes the data from the detector, and generates chromatograms for analysis. It allows for the integration and quantification of peaks, retention time determination, and data interpretation.

HPLC offers several advantages over other chromatographic techniques. It provides high sensitivity, excellent resolution, and a wide dynamic range, enabling the analysis of major and minor components in a sample. HPLC is highly versatile and can separate various compounds, from small molecules to large biomolecules. It allows for quantitative analysis by measuring peak areas or heights and can identify compounds based on retention times and spectral properties.

Different modes of HPLC are employed based on the separation requirements. RPC is the most used mode, where the stationary phase is non-polar, and the mobile phase is polar. Other modes include normal-phase chromatography, ion-exchange chromatography, size-exclusion chromatography, and chiral chromatography, each catering to specific separation needs.

HPLC is a widely utilized technique in analytical chemistry, providing precise and reliable separation and analysis of complex mixtures. Its applications range from quality control and routine analysis to research and development, making it an indispensable tool in various scientific disciplines.

Types of HPLC

Several types or modes of High-Performance Liquid Chromatography (HPLC) are designed for specific separation requirements. The choice of HPLC mode depends on the properties of the analytes and the desired separation goals. Here are some common types of HPLC:

A. Reverse-Phase Chromatography (RPC): RPC is the most widely used mode of HPLC. In this mode, the stationary phase is non-polar, typically consisting of hydrocarbon chains bonded to a solid support. In contrast, the mobile phase is polar, usually a mixture of water and an organic solvent like methanol or acetonitrile. It is suitable for separating non-polar and slightly polar compounds, such as pharmaceuticals, natural products, and lipids.

B. Normal-Phase Chromatography (NPC): Normal-phase chromatography is the reverse of RPC. Here, the stationary phase is polar, such as silica gel or alumina, while the mobile phase is non-polar, typically an organic solvent. It separates highly polar compounds, such as polar drugs, natural products, and small molecules.

C. Ion-Exchange Chromatography (IEC): IEC separates analytes based on their charge properties. The stationary phase contains ion exchange resins with charged functional groups. Positively charged analytes are attracted to the negatively charged stationary phase, while negatively charged analytes are attracted to the positively charged stationary phase. By adjusting the pH and ionic strength of the mobile phase, selective separation, and elution of charged species can be achieved.

D. Size-Exclusion Chromatography (SEC): SEC separates analytes based on size and molecular weight. The stationary phase is a porous gel or resin, and larger molecules are excluded from entering the pores and elute first, while smaller molecules penetrate the pores and elute later. It is commonly used for biomolecules, such as proteins, nucleic acids, and polysaccharides.
E. Chiral Chromatography: Chiral chromatography separates enantiomers, which are stereoisomers that are mirror images of each other. The stationary phase contains a chiral selector, a chiral small molecule, or a chiral polymer. It selectively interacts with one enantiomer, leading to differential retention and separation of the enantiomers.
F. Affinity Chromatography: Affinity chromatography utilizes the specific interaction between a target analyte and a ligand immobilized on the stationary phase. The ligand can be an antibody, enzyme, receptor, or other biomolecule. It is particularly useful for purifying and separating proteins, peptides, and other biomolecules.
G. Hydrophilic Interaction Chromatography (HILIC): HILIC combines normal-phase and RPC elements. It utilizes a polar stationary phase and a mobile phase of high organic content, resulting in retention based on the analytes' polarity. HILIC is particularly effective for separating highly polar compounds, such as polar metabolites and water-soluble vitamins.
H. Hydrophobic Interaction Chromatography (HIC): HIC is a High-Performance Liquid Chromatography (HPLC) mode that separates molecules based on their hydrophobic properties. It is a widely used technique for separating and purifying proteins, peptides, and other biomolecules.
I. Multimodal chromatography: Multimodal Chromatography also known as mixed-mode chromatography, is a chromatographic technique that combines multiple interaction mechanisms in a single stationary phase to enhance selectivity and separation

capabilities. It involves using a stationary phase that contains ligands or functional groups with different modes of interaction, such as hydrophobic, ion exchange, metal affinity, or hydrogen bonding interactions.

It's important to note that these modes of HPLC are not mutually exclusive, and multiple modes can be combined to achieve specific separation goals or enhance selectivity and resolution in complex sample mixtures. The selection of the appropriate mode depends on the nature of the analytes and the specific separation requirements.

A. Reverse-Phase Chromatography

Introduction

RPC is a widely used liquid chromatography mode that separates analytes based on their hydrophobicity or lipophilicity. It is one of the most common and versatile techniques in analytical chemistry, particularly in pharmaceutical, biotechnology, and chemical analysis.

In RPC, the stationary phase is non-polar, typically consisting of hydrocarbon chains or bonded hydrocarbons on a solid support, such as silica or polymer particles. Conversely, the mobile phase is polar, typically a mixture of water and an organic solvent like methanol, acetonitrile, or a combination of both. The mobile phase composition is varied to achieve the desired separation.

The separation mechanism in RPC is based on the differential partitioning of analytes between the hydrophobic stationary phase and the polar mobile phase. Compounds with higher hydrophobicity have stronger interactions with the hydrophobic stationary phase and are retained longer, while compounds with lower hydrophobicity elute more quickly.

The elution order in RPC is generally the opposite of the compound's polarity. Hydrophobic compounds interact more strongly with the stationary phase and are retained longer and later, while more polar compounds elute earlier.

RPC is highly effective for separating non-polar and slightly polar compounds, such as hydrophobic organic molecules, pharmaceutical drugs, lipids, and many biomolecules. It is beneficial for analyzing drugs and drug metabolites in pharmaceutical research and the analysis of proteins, peptides, and nucleic acids in biochemistry and biotechnology.

The separation selectivity in reverse-phase chromatography can be further adjusted by modifying the composition of the mobile phase. The ratio of water to organic solvent, pH, and the type and concentration of additives, such as buffers or salts, can be optimized to achieve the desired separation.

RPC is commonly performed using HPLC systems with UV-Visible or other specific detectors such as mass spectrometers. The chromatographic data generated during the analysis provides information on analyte identification, quantification, and purity.

Overall, reverse-phase chromatography is a powerful and versatile technique that offers excellent resolution, sensitivity, and reproducibility. It is widely utilized in various research fields, quality control, and analysis due to its broad applicability and ability to separate a wide range of compounds.

Components of Reverse-Phase Chromatography

Reverse-phase chromatography (RPC) is a widely used technique in liquid chromatography for separating and analyzing compounds based on their hydrophobicity. The key components involved in reverse-phase chromatography are:

Stationary Phase: The stationary phase in reverse-phase chromatography is non-polar or hydrophobic. It typically consists of hydrocarbon chains, such as C18 (octadecyl) or C8 (octyl) bonded to a solid support, such as silica or polymer particles. The hydrophobic stationary phase provides the separation mechanism by interacting with hydrophobic analytes.

Mobile Phase: The mobile phase used in reverse-phase chromatography is typically a mixture of water and an organic solvent, such as methanol, acetonitrile, or a combination of both. The mobile phase is polar and acts as the analyte carrier through the column. The composition of the mobile phase can be varied to optimize the separation and elution of target compounds.

Pump: The pump delivers the mobile phase at a constant flow rate through the column. The flow rate is typically in the range of 0.1-2 mL/min for analytical-scale separations and can be higher for preparative-scale separations. The pump ensures consistent elution of the analytes and maintains the pressure needed for optimal column performance.

Injector: The injector introduces the sample into the mobile phase flow. It can be manual or automated, depending on the instrument setup. The sample injection volume should be optimized for good peak shape and detection sensitivity.

Column: The column is a key component of reverse-phase chromatography. It contains the hydrophobic stationary phase, packed in a stainless-steel tube or other suitable material. The column's dimensions, including length and internal diameter, impact the separation efficiency and resolution. Common column lengths range from a few centimeters to several tens of centimeters, and the internal diameter can vary from a few millimeters to several millimeters.

Detector: The detector in reverse-phase chromatography monitors the eluting compounds and generates a signal that can be analyzed. UV-Visible detectors are commonly used, which measure the absorbance of the analytes at specific wavelengths. Other detectors, such as fluorescence or mass spectrometers, can also provide additional information about the separated compounds.

Data System: The data system is responsible for acquiring and analyzing chromatographic data from the detector. It captures the chromatograms, quantifies the peaks, calculates retention times, and provides data interpretation and reporting capabilities.

The components of reverse-phase chromatography work together to separate and analyze analytes based on their hydrophobicity. The choice of stationary phase, mobile phase composition, and instrument parameters should be optimized to achieve the desired separation goals and maximize the analytical performance of the technique.

Standard Operating Procedure of Reverse-Phase Chromatography

A standard operating procedure (SOP) for RPC outlines the step-by-step process for conducting a reverse-phase chromatographic analysis. Here is a general outline of an SOP for reverse-phase chromatography:

Equipment and Instrument Preparation:

- ✓ Ensure that the HPLC system is in good working condition and properly calibrated.
- ✓ Check the integrity of the column and ensure it is compatible with the analysis.
- ✓ Prepare the mobile phase according to the specified composition and degas it to remove dissolved gases.
- ✓ Set up the detector with the appropriate wavelength and sensitivity settings.

Sample Preparation:

- ✓ Prepare the sample solution by dissolving the analytes of interest in a suitable solvent.
- ✓ Filter the sample solution using a syringe filter to remove any particulates or impurities affecting the analysis.

HPLC Basics

Column Conditioning:

- ✓ Equilibrate the column with the mobile phase to ensure optimal performance and stability.
- ✓ Typically, a conditioning step involves flushing the column with the mobile phase at a constant flow rate for a specified period.

Calibration and System Suitability:

- ✓ Perform system suitability tests to verify the performance of the chromatographic system before analysis.
- ✓ Run a calibration standard mixture to ensure accurate quantification and calibration of the detector.

Sample Injection and Analysis:

- ✓ Set the appropriate injection volume and mode (e.g., partial loop or full loop injection) based on the sample concentration and system requirements.
- ✓ Inject the sample into the chromatographic system using an automated injector or manually using a syringe.
- ✓ Initiate the chromatographic run by starting the data acquisition software.
- ✓ Monitor the chromatogram in real time, observing peak shape, resolution, and baseline stability.

Data Analysis and Interpretation:

- ✓ Analyze the chromatographic data to determine peak retention times, areas, and heights.
- ✓ Calculate the analyte concentrations or other relevant parameters using calibration curves or appropriate quantification methods.
- ✓ Verify the data quality, including peak identification and integration accuracy.

HPLC Basics

- ✓ Column Regeneration and Storage:
- ✓ After the analysis, regenerate the column according to the manufacturer's recommendations to remove any accumulated contaminants.
- ✓ Following the recommended storage conditions, store the column appropriately to maintain its integrity and performance.

Documentation and Reporting:

- ✓ Document all relevant information, including sample details, instrumental parameters, and any deviations from the standard procedure.
- ✓ Prepare a report summarizing the analysis results, including peak information, concentrations, and relevant observations or conclusions.

It is important to note that the specific details and steps in an SOP for reverse-phase chromatography may vary depending on the instrument, column, and specific analysis requirements. Therefore, it is essential to customize the SOP to the specific laboratory and analytical needs and to adhere to good laboratory practices and quality assurance guidelines.

Limitations of Reverse-Phase Chromatography

Reverse-phase chromatography (RPC) is a powerful and widely used technique for separation and analysis. However, it also has certain limitations that should be considered. Here are some common limitations of RPC:

Limited Selectivity: RPC primarily relies on the hydrophobicity of analytes for separation. While this can be advantageous for non-polar and slightly polar compounds, it may not provide sufficient selectivity for highly polar compounds or compounds with similar hydrophobicity. In such cases, additional separation techniques or modifications to the stationary phase may be required.

Limited Retention of Polar Compounds: Highly polar compounds have weak interactions with the hydrophobic stationary phase, leading to poor retention and broad peaks. This can result in lower resolution and difficulties in quantification. It may require alternative chromatographic modes or modifications to enhance the retention and separation of polar analytes.

Sample Solubility Issues: Reverse-phase chromatography is often performed in organic or water-organic solvent mixtures. This can limit the solubility of some compounds, particularly hydrophilic or polar compounds, in the mobile phase. It may require sample preparation techniques, such as derivatization or solvent exchange, to improve solubility and compatibility with the chosen mobile phase.

Potential Column Interactions: The hydrophobic stationary phase used in reverse-phase chromatography can unintentionally interact with analytes. Some compounds may interact strongly with the stationary phase, leading to irreversible adsorption or peak tailing. This can result in reduced column performance, loss of resolution, and inaccurate quantification.

Sensitivity to Matrix Effects: Reverse-phase chromatography can be sensitive to matrix effects, where co-eluting compounds or sample components can interfere with the analysis. Matrix effects can affect peak shape, retention times, and quantification accuracy. Pre-treatment techniques, such as sample cleanup or matrix matching, may be required to minimize these effects.

Column Degradation and Lifetime: Reverse-phase columns can degrade over time due to interactions with samples, impurities, or harsh mobile phase conditions. Contaminants or matrix components can build up on the column, reducing column efficiency and resolution. Regular column maintenance and replacement are necessary to maintain optimal performance.

Limited pH Range: RPC is typically performed at pH values below 7 to avoid hydrolysis of the stationary phase. This can limit the analysis of unstable compounds or undergo chemical transformations at low pH values.

Limited Separation of Stereoisomers: RPC may face challenges separating stereoisomers or chiral compounds, particularly when the hydrophobic interactions alone are insufficient for achieving enantioselectivity. Specialized chiral stationary phases or alternative chromatographic modes, such as chiral chromatography, may be necessary to separate stereoisomers effectively.

Despite these limitations, RPC remains a versatile and widely used technique due to its simplicity, robustness, and compatibility with various analytes. However, it is essential to consider these limitations and, if needed, explore alternative chromatographic approaches or modifications to overcome specific challenges in separation and analysis.

B. Normal-Phase Chromatography

Introduction

Normal phase chromatography is a chromatographic technique that separates and analyzes compounds based on their polarity. In normal phase chromatography, the stationary phase is a polar material, such as silica gel or alumina, while the mobile phase is a non-polar solvent. The separation is based on the differential affinity of analytes between the polar stationary phase and the non-polar mobile phase.

In NPC, polar analytes have a greater affinity for the polar stationary phase and tend to interact more strongly with it. As a result, polar analytes are retained on the stationary phase for a longer time, leading to slower elution. Non-polar analytes, on the other hand, have a weaker affinity for the polar stationary phase and are eluted more quickly through the column.

The separation mechanism in NPC is primarily driven by polar interactions such as dipole-dipole interactions and hydrogen bonding between the polar stationary phase and the analytes. The non-polar mobile phase, which is immiscible with the stationary phase, facilitates the movement of analytes through the column.

Common stationary phases in normal phase chromatography include bare silica gel, chemically modified silica gel, and alumina. The stationary phase's choice depends on the separation's specific requirements, such as the polarity of the analytes and the desired selectivity.

The mobile phase in NPC is typically a non-polar organic solvent or a mixture of organic solvents. Commonly used mobile-phase solvents include hexane, dichloromethane, and ethyl acetate. These solvents are chosen based on their compatibility with the analytes and the stationary phase and their elution strength.

Normal phase chromatography is particularly useful for separating non-polar and polar compounds that do not retain well on reverse-phase columns. It often separates compounds, such as polar analytes, carbohydrates, natural products, and other compounds with polar functional groups.

To summarize, normal phase chromatography utilizes polar stationary and non-polar mobile phases to separate compounds based on their polarity. The interaction between the analytes and the polar stationary phase determines their retention and elution behavior. By manipulating the stationary phase andand ase composition, a wide range of compounds can be separated and analyzed using normal phase chromatography. Some key features of NPC include:

Separation of Polar Compounds: NPC is beneficial for separating polar or highly polar compounds, such as polar organic molecules, inorganic ions, small polar molecules, and certain classes of natural products.

Elution Order: In NPC, the elution order is typically the opposite of the compound's polarity. Highly polar compounds are retained longer and elute later, while non-polar compounds elute earlier.

Sample Compatibility: NPC is compatible with various sample types, including polar and non-polar analytes. However, certain sample components, such as strongly polar or ionic species, may require special considerations or modifications to the mobile phase or column.

Chiral Separations: NPC is commonly used for chiral separations. Chiral stationary phases based on modified silica gel or other polar materials can selectively interact with enantiomers, allowing for the separation of chiral compounds.

Solvent Selection: Mobile phase solvent(s) are crucial in NPC. Non-polar organic solvents are typically used to achieve elution, but the

HPLC Basics

solvent strength and composition can be adjusted to optimize separation and elution conditions.

Components of Normal Phase Chromatography

NPC involves the separation of compounds based on their polarity using a polar stationary phase and a non-polar mobile phase. The key components involved in NPC are:

Stationary Phase: The stationary phase in NPC is polar and typically consists of solid support coated or bonded with a polar material, such as silica gel or alumina. The stationary phase provides the separation mechanism by interacting with polar analytes.

Mobile Phase: The mobile phase used in NPC is non-polar or low polarity. It typically consists of non-polar organic solvents or a mixture of organic solvents, such as hexane, heptane, ethyl acetate, or dichloromethane. The mobile phase acts as a carrier for the analytes through the column and aids in their elution.

Pump: The pump delivers the mobile phase at a constant flow rate through the column. The flow rate is typically 0.5-2 mL/min for analytical-scale separations and can be higher for preparative-scale separations. The pump ensures consistent elution of the analytes and maintains the pressure needed for optimal column performance.

Injector: The injector introduces the sample into the mobile phase flow. It can be manual or automated, depending on the instrument setup. The sample injection volume should be optimized for peak shape and detection sensitivity.

Column: The column is a key component of NPC. It contains the polar stationary phase, packed in a stainless-steel tube or other suitable material. The column's dimensions, including length and internal diameter, impact the separation efficiency and resolution. Common column lengths range from a few centimeters to several tens of centimeters, and the internal diameter can vary from a few millimeters to several millimeters.

Detector: The detector in NPC monitors the eluting compounds and generates a signal that can be analyzed. UV-Visible detectors are commonly used, which measure the absorbance of the analytes at specific wavelengths. Other types of detectors, such as refractive index or evaporative light scattering detectors, can also be employed depending on the specific requirements of the analysis.

Data System: The data system is responsible for acquiring and analyzing chromatographic data from the detector. It captures the chromatograms, quantifies the peaks, calculates retention times, and provides data interpretation and reporting capabilities.

The components of NPC work together to separate and analyze analytes based on their polarity. The choice of stationary phase, mobile phase composition, and instrument parameters should be optimized to achieve the desired separation goals and maximize the analytical performance of the technique.

Standard Operating Procedure of Normal Phase Chromatography

SOP for NPC provides a step-by-step guide for performing a typical analysis using this chromatographic technique. Here is a general outline of an SOP for normal-phase chromatography:

Equipment and Instrument Preparation:

- ✓ Ensure that the chromatographic system is in good working condition and properly calibrated.
- ✓ Check the integrity of the column and ensure it is compatible with the analysis.
- ✓ Prepare the mobile phase by selecting appropriate non-polar organic solvents or solvent mixtures.

HPLC Basics

- ✓ Set up the detector with the appropriate wavelength and sensitivity settings.

Sample Preparation:

- ✓ Prepare the sample solution by dissolving the analytes of interest in a suitable solvent compatible with the mobile and stationary phases.
- ✓ Filter the sample solution using a syringe filter to remove any particulates or impurities affecting the analysis.

Column Conditioning:

- ✓ Equilibrate the column with the mobile phase to ensure optimal performance and stability.
- ✓ Typically, a conditioning step involves flushing the column with the mobile phase at a constant flow rate for a specified period.

Calibration and System Suitability:

- ✓ Perform system suitability tests to verify the performance of the chromatographic system before analysis.
- ✓ Run a calibration standard mixture to ensure accurate quantification and calibration of the detector.

Sample Injection and Analysis:

- ✓ Set the appropriate injection volume and mode (e.g., partial loop or full loop injection) based on the sample concentration and system requirements.
- ✓ Inject the sample into the chromatographic system using an automated injector or manually using a syringe.
- ✓ Initiate the chromatographic run by starting the data acquisition software.

- ✓ Monitor the chromatogram in real time, observing peak shape, resolution, and baseline stability.

Data Analysis and Interpretation:

- ✓ Analyze the chromatographic data to determine peak retention times, areas, and heights.
- ✓ Calculate the analyte concentrations or other relevant parameters using calibration curves or appropriate quantification methods.
- ✓ Verify the data quality, including peak identification and integration accuracy.

Column Regeneration and Storage:

- ✓ After the analysis, regenerate the column according to the manufacturer's recommendations to remove any accumulated contaminants.
- ✓ Following the recommended storage conditions, store the column appropriately to maintain its integrity and performance.

Documentation and Reporting:

- ✓ Document all relevant information, including sample details, instrumental parameters, and any deviations from the standard procedure.
- ✓ Prepare a report summarizing the analysis results, including peak information, concentrations, and relevant observations or conclusions.

It is important to note that the specific details and steps in an SOP for NPC may vary depending on the instrument, column, and specific analysis requirements. Therefore, it is essential to customize the SOP to the specific laboratory and analytical needs and to adhere to good laboratory practices and quality assurance guidelines.

Limitations of Normal Phase Chromatography

NPC is a widely used technique for separating and analyzing polar compounds. However, it also has certain limitations that should be taken into consideration. Here are some common limitations of NPC:

Limited Applicability for Non-Polar Compounds: NPC most effectively separates polar compounds. Non-polar compounds have weak interactions with the polar stationary phase, resulting in poor retention and broad peaks. Reverse-phase chromatography is generally more suitable for the separation of non-polar compounds.

Sensitivity to Moisture: The polar stationary phase used in NPC is moisture sensitive. High humidity or water exposure can cause irreversible changes to the stationary phase, leading to decreased separation efficiency and performance. Care must be taken to protect the column and prevent water ingress during storage and usage.

Limited Retention of Highly Polar Compounds: In normal-phase chromatography, highly polar compounds may not retain well on the polar stationary phase. They may elute quickly and result in poor resolution or co-elution with other compounds. In such cases, alternative chromatographic techniques like IEC or HILIC may be more suitable for separating highly polar analytes.

Compatibility with Aqueous Mobile Phases: NPC typically uses non-aqueous or low-aqueous mobile phases. This can limit the separation of hydrophilic or water-soluble compounds, as they may have poor retention or elute too quickly. Methods such as reverse-phase chromatography or HILIC are better suited for analyzing highly polar or water-soluble compounds.

Matrix Interferences: NPC can be sensitive to matrix effects, where co-eluting compounds or sample components interfere with the analysis. Matrix effects can lead to peak distortion, reduced resolution, and inaccurate quantification. Proper sample preparation techniques, such as sample cleanup or matrix matching, may be necessary to minimize these effects.

Limited pH Range: NPC is typically performed at pH below 7 to avoid hydrolysis or degradation of the polar stationary phase. This can limit the analysis of unstable compounds or undergo chemical transformations at low pH values. In such cases, alternative chromatographic modes or modified stationary phases may be required.

Chiral Separations: NPC alone may not be sufficient for chiral separations. While chiral stationary phases can be used, they may have limited selectivity and resolution for certain enantiomeric separations. Chiral chromatography techniques or other chiral separation methods may be more appropriate for effectively separating enantiomers.

Column Lifetime and Maintenance: Normal phase columns can be degraded due to interactions with samples, impurities, or harsh mobile phase conditions. Contaminants or matrix components can accumulate on the column, decreasing separation efficiency and performance. Regular column maintenance and replacement are necessary to maintain optimal performance.

Despite these limitations, NPC remains a valuable technique for separating and analyzing polar compounds. By understanding these limitations and exploring alternative chromatographic approaches, researchers can overcome challenges and achieve successful separations in their analyses when necessary.

C. Ion-Exchange Chromatography

Introduction

IEC is a chromatographic technique that separates and purifies charged molecules based on their interactions with charged stationary phases. It is particularly useful for separating ions, polar compounds, and biomolecules such as proteins, peptides, nucleic acids, and carbohydrates.

The principle of IEC relies on the reversible exchange of ions between the sample components in the mobile phase and the charged functional groups attached to the stationary phase. The stationary phase typically consists of a solid support, such as a resin or gel, functionalized with charged groups.

There are two main types of IEC:

Cation-Exchange Chromatography: The stationary phase contains negatively charged functional groups, such as sulfonic acid (SO_3-) or carboxylic acid ($COO-$). These negatively charged groups attract and retain positively charged ions or molecules in the sample. The mobile phase typically consists of an aqueous buffer with a pH above the pKa of the analytes, which ensures their ionization and interaction with the stationary phase.

Anion-Exchange Chromatography: The stationary phase contains positively charged functional groups, such as quaternary ammonium (NR_4+) or primary amine (NH_2+). These positively charged groups attract and retain negatively charged ions or molecules in the sample. The mobile phase typically consists of an aqueous buffer with a pH below the pKa of the analytes, promoting their ionization and interaction with the stationary phase.

The separation process in IEC involves several steps:

Column Equilibration: The column is equilibrated with the mobile phase to establish the appropriate pH and ionic strength conditions for ion-exchange interactions.

Sample Loading: The sample, typically dissolved or suspended in a suitable buffer, is injected onto the column. The charged analytes interact with the stationary phase based on their opposite charges.

Washing: Unbound or weakly bound sample components are washed away by passing the mobile phase through the column. This step removes unwanted substances and improves the purity of the target analytes.

Elution: The bound analytes are selectively eluted from the column by altering the composition of the mobile phase. This can be achieved by changing the pH, and ionic strength, or using gradient elution. The eluted analytes are collected and can be further analyzed or processed.

Regeneration: After the analysis, the column may need to be regenerated to remove any residual sample components or contaminants. This involves washing the column with appropriate solvents or buffers to restore its performance for subsequent runs.

The success of IEC depends on various factors, including the choice of stationary phase, mobile phase composition, pH, ionic strength, and temperature. It is essential to optimize these parameters to achieve the desired separation and resolution of the target analytes.

IEC finds applications in various fields, including biochemistry, pharmaceuticals, environmental analysis, food and beverage, and research laboratories. It offers a powerful tool for purifying and analyzing charged compounds, facilitating research, quality control, and process development in many industries.

Components of Ion-exchange Chromatography

IEC is a chromatographic technique used to separate and purify charged molecules. The key components involved in IEC include:

Stationary Phase: The stationary phase is a solid support material, such as resin or gel, that contains charged functional groups. These functional groups are responsible for the ion-exchange interactions with the sample components. In cation-exchange chromatography, the functional groups are negatively charged (e.g., sulfonic acid or carboxylic acid groups). In contrast, in anion-exchange chromatography, the functional groups are positively charged (e.g., quaternary ammonium or primary amine groups). The choice of stationary phase depends on the type of ions or molecules to be separated.

Mobile Phase: The mobile phase is liquid and carries the sample components through the column. It typically consists of an aqueous buffer solution that provides the necessary pH and ionic strength conditions for ion-exchange interactions. The composition of the mobile phase can be adjusted to control the elution and separation of analytes.

Pump: A pump delivers the mobile phase at a constant flow rate through the column. The flow rate is an important parameter affecting the analytes' separation efficiency and resolution. Precise control of the flow rate ensures reproducible results.

Injector: The injector introduces the sample into the mobile phase flow. The sample is usually prepared in a suitable buffer solution to maintain the desired ionic conditions and prevent precipitation or incompatibility with the mobile or stationary phase.

Column: The column contains the stationary phase packed into a cylindrical tube. The stationary phase's column length, internal diameter, and particle size are critical parameters that influence the separation performance. The column should be chosen based on the specific requirements of the separation, such as analyte size, charge, and sample load.

Detector: The detector monitors the eluting compounds and generates a signal that can be analyzed. Various detectors can be used in IEC, depending on the nature of the analytes and their detection properties. Common detectors include UV-Visible detectors, conductivity detectors, and refractive index detectors.

Data Acquisition System: A data acquisition system is used to collect and process the signals from the detector. It converts the analog detector signal into a digital format and records the chromatographic data. The data can then be analyzed and interpreted for peak identification, quantification, and further analysis.

Regeneration Solutions: Regeneration solutions are used to clean and regenerate the column after each analysis. They remove any residual sample components or contaminants that may affect the performance of the column. The regeneration solutions depend on the specific stationary phase and can include solutions of acids, bases, or salts.

Each component plays a crucial role in successfully implementing IEC. Scientists can efficiently separate and purify charged molecules in various applications by carefully selecting and optimizing these components.

Standard Operating Procedure for Ion Exchange Chromatography

Here is a general SOP for IEC:

Preparation:

- ✓ Ensure that the ion exchange column is clean and in good condition. If necessary, perform column conditioning as per the manufacturer's instructions.
- ✓ Prepare the mobile phase by accurately measuring and mixing the appropriate buffer solution to the desired pH and ionic strength.
- ✓ Check and calibrate the detectors, if required, before starting the analysis.
- ✓ Prepare the sample by dissolving or suspending it in a suitable buffer solution at the desired concentration.

Column Equilibration:

- ✓ Connect the column to the chromatographic system and ensure proper connections.
- ✓ Start the pump and equilibrate the column with the mobile phase at a specified flow rate for a sufficient period to stabilize the system (e.g., 30 minutes).
- ✓ Monitor the baseline to ensure it is stable and free from interference or drift.

Sample Loading:

- ✓ Inject a suitable volume of the prepared sample onto the column using an appropriate injection technique (e.g., loop injection or direct injection).
- ✓ Monitor the elution profile to ensure the sample components are retained on the column.

Washing:

- ✓ After the sample loading, wash the column with the mobile phase to remove unbound or weakly bound sample components.

- ✓ Monitor the elution profile and continue washing until the baseline stabilizes and unwanted components are removed.

Elution:

- ✓ Adjust the mobile phase composition or gradient program to elute the bound analytes from the column.
- ✓ Monitor the elution profile and collect fractions based on the desired retention time or peak separation.
- ✓ Record the elution time and corresponding data for each analyte.

Regeneration:

- ✓ After the analysis, regenerate the column to remove contaminants or remaining sample components.
- ✓ Flush the column with appropriate regeneration solutions as recommended by the manufacturer.
- ✓ Rinse the column with the mobile phase to ensure the complete removal of the regeneration solution.

Cleaning and Shutdown:

- ✓ Clean the column with suitable solutions to remove contaminants or residues.
- ✓ Flush the column with the mobile phase and store it according to the manufacturer's instructions.
- ✓ Shut down the chromatographic system, ensuring proper disposal of waste materials.

This is a general SOP for IEC, and specific details may vary depending on the instrument, column, and sample being analyzed. It is important to refer to the instrument manufacturer's guidelines and adapt the SOP accordingly for your specific setup. Additionally, safety precautions, waste disposal guidelines, and any specific requirements of your laboratory should be followed throughout the procedure.

Limitations of Ion-exchange Chromatography

IEC has several limitations that should be considered when using this technique:

Limited Selectivity: IEC primarily separates analytes based on their charge properties. It may not provide sufficient selectivity for samples containing closely related compounds with similar charges. Additional separation techniques or methods may be required to achieve adequate resolution.

Sample Compatibility: Some analytes may not be compatible with the ion-exchange stationery or mobile phase conditions. For example, proteins or biomolecules sensitive to high salt concentrations, extreme pH values, or harsh elution conditions may undergo denaturation or degradation during the analysis.

Limited Dynamic Range: IEC may have limitations regarding the dynamic range of sample concentrations that can be effectively analyzed. At high sample concentrations, saturation effects may occur, reducing separation efficiency and resolution.

Non-specific Binding: Non-specific binding can occur in IEC, where analytes with weak or non-specific interactions with the stationary phase may exhibit some retention level. This can lead to reduced selectivity and increased background noise in the chromatogram.

Column Fouling and Degradation: The stationary phase in IEC can become fouled or degraded over time due to the accumulation of impurities, sample residues, or irreversible interactions. This can result in decreased column performance, loss of resolution, and the need for more frequent column regeneration or replacement.

Limited Compatibility with Organic Solvents: IEC is typically performed in aqueous-based mobile phases. It may not be compatible with organic solvents, limiting its applicability to certain compounds or samples requiring organic solvents for solubility or stability.

Limited pH Range: The pH range in IEC is restricted by the stability and ionization properties of the stationary phase and the sample components. Extreme pH values may cause degradation of the stationary phase or alter the charge properties of the analytes, leading to poor separation.

Ion Suppression or Masking: In complex sample matrices, certain ions or compounds can suppress or mask the ion-exchange interactions, affecting the retention and separation of target analytes. This can result in reduced sensitivity and accuracy in the analysis.

Despite these limitations, IEC remains a valuable technique for separating and purifying charged molecules in various fields, such as biochemistry, pharmaceuticals, and environmental analysis. By understanding these limitations and optimizing the experimental conditions, researchers can overcome many challenges and obtain reliable results.

D. Size-Exclusion Chromatography

Introduction

SEC, also known as gel filtration chromatography or gel permeation chromatography, is a chromatographic technique used to separate and analyze molecules based on their size. It is particularly useful for separating biomolecules such as proteins, nucleic acids, polysaccharides, and synthetic polymers.

The principle of SEC is based on the differential partitioning of molecules between the stationary and mobile phases. The stationary phase consists of a porous gel or resin, commonly composed of cross-linked agarose or polymeric materials, with a range of defined pore sizes. Smaller molecules can enter the pores and are retained longer, while larger molecules cannot enter the pores and are eluted faster.

The separation process in SEC involves several steps:

Column Preparation: A column containing the stationary phase is prepared by packing porous gel or resin into a cylindrical tube. The size and properties of the stationary phase, such as pore size and composition, are chosen based on the size range of the target analytes.

Mobile Phase: A suitable solvent or buffer solution, the mobile phase, is selected based on the sample and the desired separation conditions. The mobile phase flows through the column, carrying the sample components.

Sample Loading: The sample is injected into the column. As the mobile phase flows through the porous stationary phase, smaller molecules can enter the pores and are excluded from the larger void spaces. They are therefore retained longer, resulting in a delayed elution time. Larger molecules cannot enter the pores and pass through the larger void spaces, leading to faster elution.

Elution: The elution occurs as the mobile phase flows through the column. The sample components are eluted from the column based on their size, with smaller molecules eluting later and larger molecules eluting earlier. This separation is achieved without specific chemical interactions between the analytes and the stationary phase.

Detection and Data Analysis: The eluted compounds are detected by suitable detectors, such as UV-Visible detectors, refractive index detectors, or light-scattering detectors. The resulting signals are recorded and analyzed to determine the retention times and peak areas, which provide information about the sample components' relative size or molecular weight.

SEC offers several advantages, including simplicity, gentle separation conditions, and compatibility with various samples. It can provide information about the distribution of molecular sizes within a sample and can be used to determine molecular weight or size exclusion limits. It is widely used in various fields, including biochemistry, biotechnology, polymer chemistry, and pharmaceutical analysis.

Components of Size-Exclusion Chromatography

SEC involves several components that work together to separate and analyze molecules based on size. The key components of SEC include:

Stationary Phase: The stationary phase is a porous gel or resin packed into a column. The stationary phase consists of cross-linked agarose or polymeric materials with defined pore sizes. The pores allow the mobile phase and sample components to enter and diffuse, leading to the separation based on size. The choice of stationary phase depends on the desired separation range and compatibility with the sample.

Mobile Phase: The mobile phase is a suitable solvent or buffer solution that carries the sample components through the column. The mobile phase does not interact specifically with the analytes based on their size but serves to transport them through the column. The composition of the mobile phase is determined based on the sample's solubility and compatibility with the stationary phase.

Column: The column is the physical structure that holds the stationary phase. It is typically a cylindrical tube made of glass or stainless steel. The column's dimensions, including length and diameter, influence the separation efficiency and capacity. The choice of column size depends on the sample volume and the resolution requirements.

Pump: A pump delivers the mobile phase at a constant flow rate through the column. The flow rate is a critical parameter affecting separation efficiency and resolution. Precise control of the flow rate ensures reproducible results.

Injector: The injector is responsible for introducing the sample into the mobile phase flow. The sample is typically dissolved or suspended in a suitable solvent or buffer to maintain the stability and solubility of the analytes. The injector can be manual or automated, depending on the system setup.

Detectors: Various detectors can be used in SEC to monitor and detect eluted compounds. Common detectors include UV-Visible detectors, refractive index detectors, and light-scattering detectors. The choice of the detector depends on the nature of the analytes and the information required from the analysis.

Data Acquisition System: A data acquisition system is used to collect and process the signals from the detector. It converts the analog detector signal into a digital format and records the chromatographic data. The data can then be analyzed and interpreted for peak identification, quantification, and further analysis.

The interaction between these components enables the separation of molecules based on their size in SEC. The stationary phase acts as a sieve, allowing smaller molecules to enter the pores and be retained longer, while larger molecules pass through the larger void spaces and elute faster. SEC can provide valuable information about the sample components' molecular weight distribution and size by carefully selecting the stationary phase, mobile phase, and operating conditions.

Standard Operating Procedure of Size-Exclusion Chromatography

A standard operating procedure (SOP) for SEC outlines the step-by-step instructions for the successful execution of the technique. Here is a generalized SOP for SEC:

Column Preparation:

- ✓ Assemble the column according to the manufacturer's instructions, ensuring proper connections.
- ✓ Equilibrate the column with the desired mobile phase by flowing it through the column at a specified flow rate for a sufficient period (e.g., 30 minutes) to remove air bubbles and stabilize the system.

Calibration of the System:

- ✓ Perform system calibration using standard reference compounds of known molecular weights.
- ✓ Inject the standard compounds into the SEC system and record their retention times and molecular weights.
- ✓ Use the calibration data to generate a calibration curve relating retention time to molecular weight.

Sample Preparation:

- ✓ Prepare the sample by dissolving or suspending it in a suitable solvent or buffer compatible with the mobile phase.
- ✓ Ensure the sample is properly filtered to remove any particulates that could interfere with the column or detector.

Sample Loading:

- ✓ Set the flow rate to the desired value according to the column specifications and system requirements.
- ✓ Inject an appropriate volume of the prepared sample onto the column using the injector, ensuring the injection is precise and reproducible.

Elution:

- ✓ Start the mobile phase flow at the specified flow rate.
- ✓ Monitor the elution of sample components using the chosen detector(s), recording the chromatographic signals (e.g., absorbance, refractive index).
- ✓ Collect eluted fractions for further analysis if necessary.

Data Analysis:

- ✓ Process the chromatographic data using appropriate software or tools.
- ✓ Determine the retention times and corresponding peak areas of the sample components.
- ✓ Use the calibration curve obtained during system calibration to estimate the molecular weights or size of the sample components.
- ✓ Perform any additional data analysis or calculations as required.

Column Regeneration and Storage:

- ✓ After completing the SEC run, regenerate the column by washing it with appropriate cleaning solutions following the manufacturer's instructions.
- ✓ Store the column according to the recommended conditions to maintain its integrity and prolong its lifespan.

It is important to note that the specific details and parameters of the SOP may vary depending on the equipment, column, and sample characteristics. Therefore, referring to the instrument manufacturer's guidelines and adapting the SOP for your specific SEC system and samples is recommended.

Limitations of Size-Exclusion Chromatography

SEC has several limitations that should be considered when choosing this technique for separation and analysis:

Resolution Limitations: SEC's resolution is generally lower than other chromatographic techniques, such as high-performance liquid chromatography (HPLC). This is because the separation in SEC is primarily based on the size of the molecules, and other factors like shape, charge, and hydrophobicity have minimal influence. As a result, molecules with similar sizes may not be well resolved.

Sample Retention Time: In SEC, smaller molecules tend to spend more time within the pores of the stationary phase, resulting in longer retention times. This can be problematic when analyzing large molecular weight samples as the elution time may be prolonged, leading to a loss of separation efficiency and increased analysis time.

Molecular Weight Determination: Although SEC provides relative size information, it does not directly measure the molecular weight of the analytes. SEC must be calibrated using standards of known molecular weights to determine the molecular weight accurately. However, calibration curves may not be linear across a broad molecular weight range, and accurate calibration for complex mixtures can be challenging.

Sample Size Requirements: SEC typically requires a relatively large sample size due to loading enough samples onto the column. This can be a limitation when working with limited sample quantities or when analyzing costly or difficult-to-obtain samples.

Limited Separation of Small Molecules: SEC is not suitable for the separation of small molecules, such as small organic compounds, ions, or small peptides. These molecules may not interact effectively with the porous stationary phase, leading to poor resolution and co-elution.

Pressure Limitations: Using porous stationary phases in SEC can result in higher backpressure, especially when working with smaller particle sizes or high flow rates. This may require specialized high-pressure systems and can limit compatibility with certain chromatographic instruments.

Limited Versatility: While SEC is widely used for separating biomolecules and polymers, it may not be suitable for all types of analytes. Complex mixtures, samples with a wide range of molecular weights, or those containing components of similar sizes may be challenging to separate effectively using SEC alone.

Despite these limitations, SEC remains a valuable tool for separating and analyzing biomolecules and polymers based on their size. It is particularly useful for characterizing macromolecular samples, determining molecular weight distributions, and assessing the purity and aggregation state of proteins and other large molecules.

E. Chiral Chromatography

Introduction

Chiral chromatography is a specialized technique used to separate and analyze enantiomers, molecules that exist as non-superimposable mirror images of each other. Enantiomers have the same chemical formula and connectivity but differ in spatial arrangement. They exhibit different biological, pharmacological, and chemical properties, making their separation and analysis crucial in various fields, particularly in the pharmaceutical and agrochemical industries.

"Chiral" refers to an object that is not superimposable on its mirror image. In chiral chromatography, the separation is achieved by exploiting the differential interaction of enantiomers with a chiral stationary phase. The chiral stationary phase is a component of the chromatographic system that possesses chirality, meaning it has a non-superimposable mirror image. The enantiomers interact differently with the chiral stationary phase, leading to their separation based on their stereochemical differences.

Chiral chromatography can be performed using different chromatographic techniques, including:

High-Performance Liquid Chromatography (HPLC): Chiral HPLC involves using a chiral stationary phase, such as chiral columns or additives, to separate enantiomers. The enantiomers are eluted at different rates based on their interactions with the stationary phase, resulting in distinct chromatographic peaks.

Gas Chromatography (GC): Chiral GC utilizes a chiral stationary phase coated on the inner wall of the GC column. Enantiomers interact differently with the stationary phase, leading to differential retention and separation.

Supercritical Fluid Chromatography (SFC): Chiral SFC combines the principles of both HPLC and GC, using a chiral stationary phase and a supercritical fluid as the mobile phase. It provides efficient separation of enantiomers with faster analysis times.

The choice of the chiral stationary phase and mobile phase depends on the specific requirements of the separation, such as the nature of the enantiomers, the sample matrix, and the desired resolution. The selector selectors used in the stationary phase can include chiral ligands, chiral polymers, chiral cyclodextrins, or chiral crown ethers.

Chiral chromatography offers several advantages, including the ability to separate enantiomers that other analytical techniques cannot differentiate. It enables the determination of enantiomeric purity, the study of chiral recognition mechanisms, and the analysis of chiral compounds in complex mixtures. Chiral chromatography plays a vital role in drug development, chiral synthesis, quality control of pharmaceuticals, and understanding the pharmacokinetics and pharmacodynamics of chiral drugs.

Components of Chiral Chromatography

Chiral chromatography involves several key components that separate and analyze enantiomers. The main components of chiral chromatography include:

Chiral Stationary Phase: The chiral stationary phase is the most critical component of chiral chromatography. It is a material or coating with chirality, meaning it has a non-superimposable mirror image. The chiral stationary phase interacts selectively with enantiomers, leading to their separation based on their stereochemical differences. Common chiral stationary phases include chiral columns, chiral additives, chiral polpolymers,rins, and chiral ligands.

Mobile Phase: The mobile phase is the solvent or mixture of solvents that carries the sample through the chiral chromatography system. The choice of mobile phase depends on the nature of the analyte and the chiral stationary phase. It should be compatible with the stationary phase and provide sufficient solubility and stability for the enantiomers. The mobile phase composition, pH, and temperature can influence the separation efficiency and selectivity.

Column: The column is the physical structure that contains the chiral stationary phase. It can be a packed column (in the case of HPLC or SFC) or a capillary column (in the case of GC). The column dimensions, such as length and internal diameter, affect the separation efficiency and resolution. The choice of the column depends on the specific application, the sample matrix, and the desired separation characteristics.

Injector: The injector introduces the sample into the chiral chromatography system. The sample should be properly prepared and dissolved or suspended in a compatible solvent to maintain the stability and solubility of the enantiomers. The injector can be manual or automated, depending on the system setup.

Detectors: Various detectors can be used in chiral chromatography to monitor and detect eluted compounds. Common detectors include UV-Visible detectors, fluorescence detectors, and mass spectrometers. The choice of detector depends on the specific application and the desired detection sensitivity and selectivity.

Data Acquisition and Analysis: A data acquisition system is used to collect and process the signals from the detector. The resulting chromatographic data is analyzed to determine the enantiomers' retention times and peak areas. Quanti Enantiomeric purity and separation efficiency assessment can be quantified appropriate software or tools.

The successful integration of these components allows for the separation and analysis of enantiomers in chiral chromatography. It is important to select and optimize these components based on the specific requirements of the analysis, including the nature of the enantiomers, sample matrix, desired resolution, and detection sensitivity.

Standard Operating Procedure of Chiral Chromatography

A standard operating procedure (SOP) for chiral chromatography provides step-by-step instructions for the proper execution of the technique. Here is a generalized SOP for chiral chromatography:

Column Preparation:

- ✓ Assemble the chiral column according to the manufacturer's instructions, ensuring proper connections.
- ✓ Equilibrate the column with the desired mobile phase by flowing it through the column at a specified flow rate for a sufficient period (e.g., 30 minutes) to remove air bubbles and stabilize the system.

Calibration of the System:

- ✓ Perform system calibration using standard reference compounds of known enantiomeric composition.
- ✓ Inject the standard compounds into the chiral chromatography system and record their retention times and corresponding enantiomeric composition.
- ✓ Use the calibration data to establish the relationship between retention times and enantiomeric composition.

Sample Preparation:

- ✓ Prepare the sample by dissolving or suspending it in a suitable solvent or mobile phase compatible with the chiral stationary phase.
- ✓ Ensure that the sample is properly filtered to remove any particulates that could interfere with the column or detector.

Mobile Phase Preparation:

- ✓ Prepare the mobile phase by mixing the appropriate solvents in the desired composition and pH, if necessary.
- ✓ Degas the mobile phase using a vacuum or inert gas to remove dissolved gases that could affect the chromatographic performance.

Instrument Setup:

- ✓ Set the appropriate flow rate, temperature, and other instrumental parameters based on the chiral column and mobile phase requirements.
- ✓ Verify the proper functioning of the injector, detector, and data acquisition system.

Sample Loading:

- ✓ Set the flow rate to the desired value according to the column specifications and system requirements.
- ✓ Inject an appropriate volume of the prepared sample onto the chiral column using the injector, ensuring that the injection is precise and reproducible.

Elution:

- ✓ Start the mobile phase flow at the specified flow rate.

- ✓ Monitor the elution of sample components using the chosen detector(s), recording the chromatographic signals (e.g., absorbance, fluorescence).
- ✓ Collect eluted fractions for further analysis if necessary.

Data Analysis:

- ✓ Process the chromatographic data using appropriate software or tools.
- ✓ Determine the retention times and peak areas of the enantiomers.
- ✓ Use the calibration curve obtained during system calibration to determine the enantiomeric composition of the sample components.
- ✓ Perform any additional data analysis or calculations as required.

Column Regeneration and Storage:

- ✓ After completing the chiral chromatography run, regenerate the column by washing it with appropriate cleaning solutions following the manufacturer's instructions.
- ✓ Store the column according to the recommended conditions to maintain its integrity and prolong its lifespan.

It is important to note that the specific details and parameters of the SOP may vary depending on the equipment, column, sample characteristics, and specific chiral separation method employed (HPLC, GC, SFC). Therefore, it is recommended to refer to the instrument manufacturer's guidelines and adapt the SOP accordingly for your specific chiral chromatography system and samples.

Limitations of Chiral Chromatography

Despite its effectiveness in separating and analyzing enantiomers, chiral chromatography has certain limitations that should be considered. Some of the limitations of chiral chromatography include:

Limited Availability of Chiral Stationary Phases: Chiral stationary phases are crucial for chiral chromatography, and a wide range of chiral selectors can be limited. The availability may vary depending on the desired separation mechanism (e.g., reversed-phase, normal-phase, ion exchange) and the specific analytes of interest. The lack of suitable chiral stationary phases for certain enantiomers or compounds can restrict the application of chiral chromatography.

Separation Efficiency: Chiral chromatography may face challenges in achieving high separation efficiency, especially for complex mixtures. Some enantiomers may exhibit similar interactions with the chiral stationary phase, resulting in poor resolution and co-elution. This can make the quantification and analysis of individual enantiomers challenging. Additional optimization steps, such as modifying the mobile phase composition or column conditions, may be required to improve separation efficiency.

Sample Compatibility: Chiral chromatography requires samples to be soluble and compatible with the chosen mobile and chiral stationary phases. Some compounds, particularly those with limited solubility or high reactivity, may not be suitable for chiral chromatography analysis. Incompatibility issues can result in peak broadening, poor resolution, or irreversible interactions with the stationary phase, leading to inaccurate or unreliable results.

Method Development Complexity: Developing a chiral chromatography method can be more complex compared to achiral chromatography. The selection of an appropriate chiral stationary phase, optimization of the mobile phase composition, and establishment of separation conditions may require extensive method development and screening. This process can be time-consuming and resource intensive.

Cost: Chiral chromatography can be more expensive than achiral chromatography. Chiral stationary phases and columns may be more costly due to their specialized nature and limited availability. Moreover, chiral chromatography may require more frequent column regeneration and replacement due to fouling or degradation of the chiral stationary phase.

Lack of Universal Method: Chiral chromatography methods are often specific to chiral selectors and applications. There is no universal method that can separate all types of enantiomers effectively. Method development may need to be tailored to individual analytes or classes of compounds, which can limit the general applicability of a single method.

Despite these limitations, chiral chromatography remains a powerful tool for enantiomeric separation and analysis. Advancements in chiral stationary phase development, method optimization, and technology continue to address these limitations and expand the utility of chiral chromatography in various fields such as pharmaceuticals, agrochemicals, and natural product analysis.

F. Affinity Chromatography

Introduction

Affinity chromatography is a separation technique used to purify and isolate specific biomolecules based on their specific binding interactions with a complementary ligand or ligand binder. It is commonly employed in various fields, such as biochemistry, biotechnology, and pharmaceutical research.

The principle of affinity chromatography is based on the affinity or specific binding between a target molecule (analyte) and a ligand binder (affinity ligand) immobilized on a solid support. The target molecule may be a protein, enzyme, antibody, nucleic acid, or any other biomolecule of interest.

The general steps involved in affinity chromatography are as follows:

Ligand Immobilization: The ligand binder is covalently attached or immobilized onto a solid support material, such as agarose beads, magnetic particles, or chromatographic resin. The immobilization method may involve chemical cross-linking, affinity tags, or other techniques, depending on the nature of the ligand binder and the support material.

Sample Preparation: The sample containing the target molecule is prepared by removing impurities, such as cell debris or other contaminants, through various pre-treatment steps like cell lysis, filtration, or centrifugation. The sample is usually dissolved or suspended in a suitable buffer or mobile phase compatible with the affinity chromatography system.

Column Preparation: The affinity chromatography column is packed with the immobilized ligand binder. The column dimensions and the amount of ligand binder depend on the desired binding capacity and resolution.

Binding and Washing: The prepared sample is loaded onto the affinity column, and the target molecule selectively binds to the immobilized ligand binder due to specific binding interactions. The non-specific or unbound molecules are washed away using a suitable buffer or wash solution to remove contaminants and unwanted components.

Elution: The bound target molecule is selectively eluted from the affinity column using elution buffers or conditions that disrupt the binding interactions. The elution can be achieved by changing the pH, ionic strength, or temperature or by using competitive ligands that outcompete the target molecule for binding to the ligand binder.

Analysis and Purification: The eluted fractions containing the purified target molecule are collected and analyzed using appropriate techniques such as gel electrophoresis, mass spectrometry, or enzymatic assays. Further purification steps may be performed depending on the specific requirements of the downstream application.

Affinity chromatography offers several advantages, including high specificity and selectivity for the target molecule, high binding capacity, and the ability to purify molecules from complex mixtures. It is widely used in protein purification, antibody purification, isolation of enzymes, and other biomolecules with specific binding properties.

Components of Affinity Chromatography

Affinity chromatography involves several key components that work together to facilitate the separation and purification of target molecules based on specific binding interactions. The main components of affinity chromatography include:

Ligand Binder (Affinity Ligand): The ligand binder is a molecule or compound specifically binding to the target molecule of interest. It is immobilized onto a solid support matrix, such as beads or resin, which provides a large surface area for binding interactions. The ligand binder can be an antibody, enzyme, receptor, nucleic acid, or any other molecule capable of recognizing and binding to the target molecule.

Solid Support Matrix: The solid support matrix serves as the stationary phase in affinity chromatography. It can be composed of various materials, such as agarose, cellulose, or magnetic particles, that are chemically modified to allow immobilization of the ligand binder. The choice of the support matrix depends on factors such as compatibility with the target molecule and the specific affinity ligand used.

Sample Loading System: The sample loading system allows the introduction of the sample into the affinity chromatography system. It typically consists of an injection port or sample loop connected to the chromatographic column. The sample should be properly prepared and dissolved or suspended in a suitable buffer or mobile phase to ensure efficient interaction with the ligand binder.

Chromatographic Column: The chromatographic column contains the immobilized ligand binder and serves as the site of separation. It is packed with the solid support matrix coated with the ligand binder, ensuring proper binding and interaction with the target molecule. The column dimensions and packing efficiency play a crucial role in achieving optimal separation and purification.

Mobile Phase: The mobile phase is a solvent or buffer system that carries the sample through the affinity chromatography system. It provides the necessary conditions for the binding interactions between the target molecule and the ligand binder. The composition and pH of the mobile phase are carefully selected to optimize the binding and elution processes.

Elution Buffer: The elution buffer is used to disrupt the specific binding interactions between the target molecule and the ligand binder, leading to the release of the target molecule from the affinity column. The elution buffer is designed to have a higher affinity for the ligand binder, allowing the target molecule to be selectively eluted while minimizing non-specific interactions.

Detector: Various detectors can be used in affinity chromatography to monitor and detect the eluted target molecule. Common detectors include UV-Visible detectors, fluorescence detectors, or mass spectrometers, depending on the nature of the target molecule and the desired detection sensitivity and selectivity.

The successful integration of these components allows for the selective separation and purification of target molecules in affinity chromatography. It is important to select the appropriate ligand binder, solid support matrix, and mobile phase conditions based on the specific characteristics of the target molecule and the intended application.

Standard Operating Procedure of Affinity Chromatography

A standard operating procedure (SOP) for affinity chromatography provides step-by-step instructions for the proper execution of the technique. Here is a generalized SOP for affinity chromatography:

Preparation of Ligand Binder and Support Matrix:

- ✓ Immobilize the ligand binder onto the solid support matrix according to the manufacturer's instructions.
- ✓ Ensure that the ligand binder is properly attached to the support matrix, and any excess or unbound ligand binder is removed.

Column Preparation:

- ✓ Assemble the affinity chromatography column, ensuring that it is clean and free from any contaminants.
- ✓ Pack the column with the ligand binder-immobilized support matrix, following the recommended packing procedure and guidelines.
- ✓ Equilibrate the column with an appropriate equilibration buffer to remove any residual contaminants and stabilize the system.

Sample Preparation:

- ✓ Prepare the sample containing the target molecule of interest by removing any particulates or contaminants through suitable pre-treatment steps such as filtration, centrifugation, or purification.
- ✓ Dissolve or suspend the sample in a compatible buffer or mobile phase that maintains the stability and integrity of the target molecule.

Mobile Phase Preparation:

- ✓ Prepare the mobile phase by selecting an appropriate buffer or solvent system that provides optimal binding and elution conditions for the ligand binder and the target molecule.
- ✓ Ensure that the mobile phase is properly degassed to remove any dissolved gases that could affect the chromatographic performance.

Column Equilibration:

- ✓ Connect the prepared affinity chromatography column to the chromatographic system.
- ✓ Equilibrate the column with the chosen mobile phase at the recommended flow rate to establish a stable baseline and remove any air bubbles.

Sample Loading:

- ✓ Load the prepared sample onto the affinity column using an injection port or sample loop, ensuring precise and reproducible sample application.
- ✓ Adjust the flow rate to the recommended value to achieve optimal interaction between the target molecule and the ligand binder.

Washing:

- ✓ Wash the column with the equilibration buffer or a suitable wash buffer to remove non-specifically bound molecules and contaminants.
- ✓ Optimize the wash conditions based on the target molecule and the affinity ligand used, ensuring effective removal of impurities while retaining the specific binding interaction.

Elution:

- ✓ Select an appropriate elution buffer or conditions that disrupt the specific binding interaction between the target molecule and the ligand binder.
- ✓ Apply the elution buffer to the column to release the target molecule from the affinity matrix.
- ✓ Collect the eluted fractions containing the purified target molecule for further analysis or downstream applications.

Column Regeneration and Storage:

- ✓ After completing the affinity chromatography run, regenerate the column by washing it with appropriate cleaning solutions following the manufacturer's guidelines.
- ✓ Store the column according to the recommended conditions to maintain its integrity and prolong its lifespan.

It is important to note that the specific details and parameters of the SOP may vary depending on the ligand binder, support matrix, target molecule, and specific affinity chromatography system employed. It is recommended to refer to the instrument manufacturer's guidelines and adapt the SOP accordingly for your specific affinity chromatography system and samples.

Limitations of Affinity Chromatography

While affinity chromatography is a powerful technique for the separation and purification of target molecules, it also has certain limitations that should be considered. Some of the limitations of affinity chromatography include:

Specificity: Affinity chromatography relies on the specific binding interactions between the ligand binder and the target molecule. The success of the technique is highly dependent on the specificity and strength of these interactions. If the affinity ligand or ligand binder is not highly specific for the target molecule, there may be challenges in achieving high purification levels and separation from closely related molecules.

Ligand Binding Capacity: The binding capacity of the affinity ligand can limit the amount of target molecule that can be loaded onto the column. If the binding capacity is low, it may require larger volumes or multiple runs to purify enough of the target molecule. This can be particularly limiting when working with low-abundance or rare target molecules.

Sample Complexity: Affinity chromatography may encounter difficulties when dealing with complex samples containing numerous components. In such cases, there may be non-specific binding of other molecules to the ligand binder, leading to decreased purity and resolution of the target molecule. Pre-treatment steps or additional purification techniques may be required to overcome these challenges.

Ligand Stability: The stability of the ligand binder, particularly when immobilized on the solid support matrix, is critical for the longevity and reproducibility of affinity chromatography. If the ligand binder loses activity or degrades over time, it can affect the performance and reliability of the purification process. Stability issues may arise due to factors such as temperature, pH, or the presence of denaturing agents.

Scale-Up Challenges: Scaling up affinity chromatography from laboratory scale to industrial scale can present challenges. The availability and cost of large quantities of ligand binders and support matrices may be limiting factors. Additionally, the process of packing large columns with consistent and reproducible results can be challenging.

Time and Cost: Affinity chromatography can be a time-consuming and expensive technique compared to other chromatographic methods. The production and purification of the affinity ligand, as well as the immobilization of the ligand binder, can require significant resources. Furthermore, affinity chromatography may involve multiple purification steps and reagents, increasing the overall cost and time required for the process.

Ligand Regeneration: Some affinity ligands may irreversibly bind to the target molecule, making it difficult to regenerate and reuse the ligand binder. The need for frequent replacement or regeneration of the ligand binder can add to the overall cost and complexity of the purification process.

Despite these limitations, affinity chromatography remains a valuable tool for purifying and isolating specific biomolecules. Advances in ligand design, ligand immobilization techniques, and column technology continue to address these limitations and enhance the performance and applicability of affinity chromatography in various fields, including biotechnology, pharmaceuticals, and protein research.

G. Hydrophilic Interaction Chromatography

Introduction

HILIC is a chromatographic technique used to separate and analyze polar and hydrophilic compounds. It is particularly effective for the repetitioning and separating of molecules, highly hydrophilic compounds, and compounds with a wide range of polarities.

In HILIC, the stationary phase is typically a polar material such as silica or a polar-modified material. In contrast, the mobile phase consists of water-rich, polar solvents such as acetonitrile or methanol, often with a small percentage of a buffer or salt. The hydrophilic stationary phase facilitates the partitioning and retention of polar analytes, allowing for their separation based on differences in polarity, size, and other properties.

The separation mechanism in HILIC involves a combination of partitioning and adsorption interactions. The polar stationary phase can form hydrogen bonds, dipole-dipole interactions, or other polar interactions with the analytes, resulting in their differential retention and separation. Analytes with stronger hydrophilic interactions with the stationary phase will have longer retention times, while less hydrophilic or non-polar analytes will elute earlier.

HILIC has several advantages over other chromatographic techniques, such as RPC. It can effectively separate highly polar and water-soluble compounds that may not retain well in RPC. It is also useful for separating and retaining compounds with similar polarities but different chemical functionalities. HILIC is widely employed in various fields, including pharmaceutical analysis, metabolomics, proteomics, environmental analysis, and bioanalysis.

To perform HILIC, specialized HILIC columns, and appropriate mobile phase conditions are required. The column choice, mobile phase composition, pH, and other parameters will depend on the specific analytes and separation goals. Experimental optimization may be necessary to achieve the desired separation and resolution.

It is important to consult scientific literature and specialized chromatography textbooks or consult with experts to obtain more detailed information, specific applications, and advances in HILIC methodology.

Components of Hydrophilic Interaction Chromatography

HILIC typically involves several key components that contribute to the separation and analysis of polar and hydrophilic compounds. These components include:

Stationary Phase: The stationary phase used in HILIC is typically a polar material that interacts with the polar analytes. Silica-based materials with polar functional groups, such as amino or diol groups, are commonly employed. Other polar-modified stationary phases, such as zwitterionic or hydrophilic polymer-based materials, are also available. The choice of stationary phase depends on the specific separation requirements and the properties of the analytes.

Mobile Phase: The mobile phase in HILIC is typically a water-rich, polar solvent. Commonly used solvents include acetonitrile, methanol, or mixtures of water and organic solvents. Adding small amounts of buffer or salts to the mobile phase can help control the ionic strength and improve separation selectivity. The composition and pH of the mobile phase are critical parameters that influence the retention and separation of analytes in HILIC.

Sample Preparation: Sample preparation for HILIC may involve extraction or purification steps to isolate the target analytes from complex matrices. Depending on the nature of the sample, techniques such as liquid-liquid extraction, solid-phase extraction (SPE), or other sample cleanup methods may be employed.

Injection System: An appropriate injection system is required to introduce the prepared sample onto the HILIC column. Common injection techniques include manual or autosampler injections, which should be optimized to ensure reproducibility and avoid any sample degradation or contamination.

HILIC Column: HILIC columns are designed specifically for HILIC. These columns have a polar stationary phase coating or functionalization that enables the retention and separation of polar analytes. Typical column dimensions include length, internal diameter, and particle size, affecting separation efficiency, resolution, and analysis time.

Detection System: Various techniques can be employed to analyze the separated analytes. Common detection methods include UV-Vis spectroscopy, mass spectrometry (MS), evaporative light scattering detection (ELSD), refractive index detection (RID), or fluorescence detection. The choice of detection system depends on the analyte properties and the desired sensitivity and selectivity.

It's important to note that the specific components and parameters used in HILIC can vary depending on the application, target analytes, and separation goals. Therefore, it's recommended to consult scientific literature and chromatography method guides or consult with experts for detailed guidance and specific recommendations.

Standard Operating Procedure of Hydrophilic Interaction Chromatography

The standard operating procedure (SOP) for HILIC can vary depending on the specific laboratory, instrument, and application.

However, here is a general outline of the steps involved in conducting HILIC:

Instrument Preparation:

- ✓ Ensure that the HPLC or UHPLC system is in good working condition.
- ✓ Check the column and ensure it is properly installed and in good condition.
- ✓ Verify that the mobile phase reservoirs contain the appropriate solvents and that they are properly connected to the system.
- ✓ Calibrate and verify the performance of the detectors (e.g., UV-Vis, mass spectrometer) if required.

Mobile Phase Preparation:

- ✓ Prepare the HILIC mobile phase by mixing appropriate amounts of water and organic solvent (e.g., acetonitrile, methanol) based on the desired composition. Add buffer or salts, if necessary, to adjust the pH or ionic strength.
- ✓ Thoroughly mix the components to ensure proper homogeneity of the mobile phase.
- ✓ Filter the mobile phase using a suitable membrane or filter to remove any particulates or impurities.

Sample Preparation:

- ✓ Extract or purify the sample of interest using suitable techniques such as liquid-liquid extraction, solid-phase extraction (SPE), or other methods, depending on the sample matrix and analyte properties.
- ✓ Concentrate or reconstitute the extracted sample to an appropriate volume or concentration for injection.
- ✓ Filter the sample using a suitable syringe filter to remove any particulates or insoluble materials that could interfere with the HILIC analysis.

Column Conditioning:

- ✓ Equilibrate the HILIC column with the mobile phase before analysis.
- ✓ Follow the manufacturer's recommendations regarding the column equilibration procedure, including the duration and flow rate of the mobile phase.

Injection and Analysis:

- ✓ Set the appropriate injection volume, typically in microliters (µL), depending on the sample concentration and instrument capabilities.
- ✓ Inject the prepared sample onto the equilibrated HILIC column using the selected injection method (e.g., manual injection, autosampler).
- ✓ Initiate the chromatographic run with the predefined method parameters, including column temperature, flow rate, and gradient conditions if applicable.
- ✓ Monitor the separation progress using the selected detection system (e.g., UV-Vis, mass spectrometer) and adjust parameters if necessary.

Data Analysis and Interpretation:

- ✓ Collect and analyze the chromatographic data obtained during the HILIC analysis.
- ✓ Identify and quantify the analytes of interest based on their retention times, peak shapes, and spectral properties.
- ✓ Interpret the chromatographic results, including peak identification, integration, and calculation of analyte concentrations or other relevant parameters.

Post-Analysis:

- ✓ Properly dispose of waste materials generated during the HILIC analysis, following the established laboratory protocols and safety guidelines.
- ✓ Clean and maintain the HPLC/UHPLC system and the HILIC column according to the manufacturer's recommendations.

It's important to note that the SOP for HILIC may be specific to each laboratory or analytical method. It's recommended to consult with your laboratory's standard operating procedures, instrument manuals, or experts in the field for detailed instructions tailored to your specific setup and requirements.

Limitations of Hydrophilic Interaction Chromatography

HILIC has several advantages for separating polar and hydrophilic compounds, but it also has certain limitations. Here are some common limitations of HILIC:

Limited Retention Time Range: HILIC is most effective for separating highly polar and hydrophilic compounds. However, it may not retain analytes with very low polarity or non-polar compounds as effectively as other chromatographic techniques, such as reversed-phase chromatography (RPC). This limited retention range can make achieving optimal separation for analytes with a wide range of polarities challenging.

Sensitivity to Mobile Phase Composition: The separation and retention in HILIC strongly depend on the composition and properties of the mobile phase. Small changes in the mobile phase composition, such as altering the water content, pH, or buffer concentration, can significantly affect the selectivity and elution behavior of analytes. This sensitivity requires careful optimization of the mobile phase conditions for each specific application.

Limited Column Lifetimes: HILIC columns can experience a shorter life than those used in other chromatographic techniques. The polar stationary phase can be prone to fouling and irreversible adsorption of polar compounds, resulting in reduced column performance and increased baseline noise over time. Regular column maintenance and proper sample clean-up methods are essential to minimize these effects.

Challenging Method Development: Developing robust HILIC methods can be more challenging than other chromatographic techniques. Finding the right combination of stationary phase, mobile phase, and other method parameters to achieve the desired separation can require extensive optimization and trial and error. Method development in HILIC often involves exploring various column chemistries, mobile phase compositions, and gradient conditions.

Matrix Effects: HILIC can be sensitive to matrix effects caused by interfering compounds or co-eluting substances in complex samples. Co-elution or overlapping peaks from matrix components can hinder the detection and quantification of target analytes. Adequate sample preparation techniques, such as solid-phase extraction (SPE) or other clean-up methods, may be necessary to minimize matrix effects.

Limited Compatibility with Some Detectors: HILIC may not be compatible with certain detection techniques commonly used in other chromatographic methods. For example, refractive index detectors (RID) may not provide adequate sensitivity and selectivity in HILIC due to the low refractive index differences between the mobile phase and analytes. Alternative detection methods, such as mass spectrometry (MS), fluorescence, or UV-Vis detectors, are often preferred for HILIC analysis.

Despite these limitations, HILIC remains a valuable technique for the separation and analysis of polar and hydrophilic compounds. By understanding these limitations and proper method optimization, researchers can leverage the strengths of HILIC to achieve accurate and reliable separations in specific applications.

H. Hydrophobic Interaction Chromatography

Introduction

HIC is a chromatographic technique used for the separation and purification of biomolecules based on their hydrophobic properties. It is particularly useful for separating proteins, peptides, and nucleic acids.

Principles of HIC:

Hydrophobic interactions: HIC takes advantage of the hydrophobic interactions between the hydrophobic regions of biomolecules and hydrophobic ligands attached to the stationary phase of the chromatography column. These hydrophobic regions can be found on the surface of proteins, which may be exposed due to the folding or denaturation of the molecule.

Binding and elution: In HIC, the stationary phase of the chromatography column is typically composed of hydrophobic ligands, such as alkyl chains. When a sample containing biomolecules is applied to the column, the hydrophobic regions of the biomolecules interact with the hydrophobic ligands, leading to their retention on the column. Elution is achieved by decreasing the hydrophobicity of the mobile phase or by using a gradient of increasing polarity, which reduces the hydrophobic interactions and releases the bound molecules.

Selectivity: The selectivity of HIC can be controlled by adjusting parameters such as the nature and length of the hydrophobic ligands, pH, salt concentration, and temperature. These parameters influence the strength of the hydrophobic interactions and can be optimized to achieve the desired separation.

Applications of HIC:

HIC is widely used in various areas of bio-separation and purification, including:

Protein purification: HIC can effectively separate proteins based on their hydrophobicity, allowing the removal of impurities and isolation of the target protein.

Protein fractionation: HIC can separate different protein variants or isoforms that have slight differences in their hydrophobicity.

Viral purification: HIC can be employed in the purification of viruses and viral particles, taking advantage of the hydrophobic regions present on their surface.

Nucleic acid purification: HIC can separate and purify nucleic acids based on their hydrophobic properties, facilitating applications such as plasmid DNA purification.

HIC is a valuable tool in chromatography, offering a complementary technique to other separation methods like size exclusion chromatography, ion exchange chromatography, and affinity chromatography. By utilizing the hydrophobic characteristics of biomolecules, HIC provides a versatile approach for separating and purifying uses in various biological and biotechnological applications.

Components of Hydrophobic Interaction Chromatography

The key components of HIC include:

Stationary Phase: The stationary phase in HIC is a hydrophobic material or resin with hydrophobic functional groups. Examples of commonly used hydrophobic stationary phases include phenyl, butyl, octyl, or octadecyl groups attached to a solid support such as silica or resin beads. The hydrophobic nature of the stationary phase allows for selective retention of hydrophobic analytes.

Mobile Phase: The mobile phase in HIC is an aqueous buffer containing a high concentration of a chaotropic salt, such as ammonium sulfate or sodium chloride. The chaotropic salt disrupts the water structure and weakens the water-hydrophobic interactions, enabling the hydrophobic analytes to interact with the stationary phase. The concentration of the chaotropic salt can be adjusted to modulate the strength of the hydrophobic interactions and control the elution of analytes.

Pump: The pump is responsible for delivering the mobile phase at a constant flow rate throughout the chromatographic run. It ensures consistent and reproducible separation conditions.

Injector: The injector is used to introduce the sample onto the column. It allows for precise and controlled sample loading onto the stationary phase.

Column: The column contains the hydrophobic stationary phase where the separation of analytes occurs. The column is packed with hydrophobic resin or particles with hydrophobic functional groups. It provides the necessary surface area for analyte-stationary phase interactions.

Detector: The detector monitors the eluted compounds from the column and generates a signal that is recorded and analyzed. Various detectors can be used in HIC, including UV-Visible detectors, fluorescence detectors, or mass spectrometers, depending on the nature of the analytes and the desired detection sensitivity.

Data System: The data system or chromatography software controls the instrument, acquires, and processes data from the detector, and generates chromatograms for analysis. It allows for peak integration, quantification, and data interpretation.

These components work together to facilitate the separation and analysis of hydrophobic analytes based on their affinity for the hydrophobic stationary phase. The hydrophobic interactions between the analytes and the stationary phase drive the retention and elution of analytes, enabling their separation based on their hydrophobic properties.

Standard Operating Procedure of Hydrophobic Interaction Chromatography

SOP for HIC typically includes the following steps:

Mobile Phase Preparation:

- ✓ Prepare the mobile phase by dissolving the appropriate buffer and chaotropic salt in distilled water.
- ✓ Adjust the pH of the buffer if necessary.
- ✓ Filter the mobile phase using a suitable membrane filter to remove any particulate matter.

Column Preparation:

- ✓ Equilibrate the HIC column with the mobile phase by flushing it with the mobile phase at the desired flow rate for a sufficient duration.
- ✓ Ensure that the column is properly connected to the chromatography system.

System Equilibration:

- ✓ Prime the system by flushing it with the mobile phase to ensure that all components are filled with the mobile phase.
- ✓ Allow the system to equilibrate for a specified period to ensure stable baseline conditions.

HPLC Basics

Sample Preparation:

- ✓ Prepare the sample by dissolving the analytes of interest in an appropriate solvent or buffer compatible with the mobile phase.
- ✓ Ensure that the sample is free from particulate matter and properly filtered if necessary.

Sample Injection:

- ✓ Load an appropriate volume of the prepared sample onto the HIC column using an injector or sample loop.
- ✓ Ensure that the injection is precise and reproducible.

Gradient Elution:

- ✓ Initiate the chromatographic run by setting the desired gradient program.
- ✓ Gradually change the chaotropic salt concentration in the mobile phase according to the established gradient program.
- ✓ Monitor the elution of analytes using the selected detector(s).

Data Analysis:

- ✓ Collect and analyze the chromatographic data using suitable software.
- ✓ Analyze the peak shapes, retention times, and peak areas to determine the separation efficiency and quantify the analytes of interest.
- ✓ Perform necessary calculations and data interpretation to obtain desired results.

Column Regeneration:

- ✓ After the analysis is complete, regenerate the column by washing it with a suitable regeneration solution or mobile phase to remove any remaining sample residues or contaminants.

✓ Equilibrate the column with the initial mobile phase composition for subsequent runs.

System Shutdown:

✓ Flush the system with the appropriate solvent to clean the flow path and prevent residual salt precipitation or contamination.
✓ Ensure proper storage and maintenance of the chromatography system.

It is important to note that the specific details and parameters of the SOP may vary depending on the specific HIC system, column, analytes, and desired separation conditions. It is crucial to refer to the instrument and column manufacturer's instructions and optimize the method parameters for the specific application.

Limitations of Hydrophobic Interaction Chromatography

HIC has several limitations that should be considered:

Limited Resolution: HIC is generally less efficient in achieving high resolution than other chromatographic techniques such as reversed-phase chromatography. This is particularly true for complex samples containing closely related hydrophobic analytes, where separating might be challenging.

Sample Denaturation: In some cases, HIC can lead to sample denaturation or loss of biological activity. The interaction between hydrophobic ligands on the stationary phase and the hydrophobic regions of the analyte can disrupt the native conformation and functional properties of the biomolecules.

Limited Dynamic Range: HIC best separates analytes with moderate to high hydrophobicity. For highly hydrophilic or highly hydrophobic analytes, the separation may not be as effective, leading to poor resolution or co-elution.

Limited Selectivity: While HIC is effective for separating hydrophobic compounds, it may not provide enough selectivity for samples with analytes that have similar hydrophobicity. Additional techniques or orthogonal separation methods may be required for a more comprehensive separation.

Requirement for Optimization: HIC requires careful optimization of mobile phase conditions, including salt concentration, pH, and temperature, to achieve optimal separation. This optimization process can be time-consuming and may require significant trial and error.

Limited Compatibility with Biological Matrices: HIC may encounter challenges when dealing with complex biological samples that contain high salt concentrations or other components that can interfere with the chromatographic separation. Sample preparation steps, such as desalting or clean-up, may be necessary to overcome these challenges.

Limited Reusability: The hydrophobic stationary phase used in HIC may have limited reusability due to fouling or irreversible adsorption of sample components. This can result in reduced column performance over time and necessitate more frequent column replacement or regeneration.

Limited Availability of Stationary Phases: Compared to other chromatographic techniques, the variety of commercially available hydrophobic stationary phases for HIC might be more limited. This can restrict the flexibility and choice of stationary phases for specific separation needs.

It is important to carefully consider these limitations when deciding whether to use HIC for a particular separation or when designing chromatographic methods. Proper optimization, sample preparation, and consideration of alternative separation techniques can help mitigate some of these limitations and enhance the effectiveness of HIC.

I. Multimodal Chromatography

Introduction

Multimodal chromatography is a chromatographic technique that utilizes stationary phases with multiple interaction modes to separate and purify target molecules from complex mixtures. Unlike traditional chromatography methods that rely on a single interaction mechanism, multimodal chromatography combines multiple interactions, such as hydrophobic, ion exchange, hydrogen bonding, and affinity interactions, to achieve higher selectivity and improved purification efficiency.

In multimodal chromatography, the stationary phase is typically modified with ligands with different binding properties. These ligands can interact with the target molecule through various mechanisms, allowing for a more specific and robust separation process. The choice of ligands and the specific combination of interaction modes depend on the properties of the target molecule and the desired purification goals.

The benefits of multimodal chromatography include:

Enhanced Selectivity: By employing multiple interaction modes, multimodal chromatography offers enhanced selectivity for target molecules. It allows for the simultaneous exploitation of different physicochemical properties, separating closely related compounds or impurities that may have similar characteristics.

Increased Binding Capacity: Multimodal chromatography can provide higher binding capacities than traditional chromatography methods. The multiple interaction mechanisms enable greater interaction between the target molecule and the stationary phase, increasing adsorption and retention capacity.

Flexible Purification Strategies: With multimodal chromatography, purification strategies can be tailored and optimized based on the specific requirements of the target molecule. The choice of ligands and operating conditions can be adjusted to achieve the desired selectivity and purification efficiency, making it a versatile technique for various applications.

Reduced Process Complexity: Multimodal chromatography can streamline purification processes by reducing the required steps and unit operations. It eliminates the need for multiple chromatography steps using different separation modes, simplifying the overall process, and reducing the time and cost associated with purification.

Compatibility with Complex Feedstocks: Multimodal chromatography is suitable for purifying complex feedstocks that contain a mixture of target molecules and impurities. It can effectively handle crude samples, such as cell lysates or fermentation broths, and selectively capture and purify the desired molecules while removing impurities.

Purification of Fragile Biomolecules: Multimodal chromatography also applies to purifying delicate biomolecules, including proteins, antibodies, enzymes, and nucleic acids. The flexibility of the technique allows for gentle purification conditions, preserving the integrity and functionality of the biomolecules during the purification process.

Multimodal chromatography has applications in various fields, including biopharmaceutical manufacturing, protein purification, natural product isolation, and analytical chemistry. It is a valuable tool for achieving high-resolution separations, purifying complex mixtures, and obtaining purified target molecules with improved yield and purity.

Components of Multimodal Chromatography

Multimodal chromatography utilizes stationary phases with multiple interaction modes to achieve enhanced selectivity in the separation and purification of target molecules. The components involved in multimodal chromatography can vary depending on the specific implementation and the desired separation goals. However, there are several common components typically found in multimodal chromatography systems:

Stationary Phase: The stationary phase is a crucial component in multimodal chromatography. It consists of solid support material, such as beads or membranes, onto which ligands with different interaction modes are immobilized. These ligands provide the multiple interaction mechanisms required for the enhanced selectivity of the chromatographic process.

Ligands: Ligands are chemical entities attached to the stationary phase that facilitate the interactions between the target molecules and the stationary phase. Ligands with different functional groups and interaction modes are used in multimodal chromatography to achieve multiple interaction mechanisms. Examples of ligands commonly employed in multimodal chromatography include hydrophobic groups, ion-exchange groups, affinity ligands, and hydrogen bonding groups.

Mobile Phase: The mobile phase is a solvent or buffer that carries the sample through the chromatographic system. It plays a crucial role in eluting the target molecules from the stationary phase based on the desired separation conditions. The composition and pH of the mobile phase can be adjusted to modulate the interactions between the target molecules and the stationary phase.

Chromatography Columns: Chromatography columns contain the stationary phase and facilitate the separation process. The columns can be packed with beads or contain membranes coated with ligands. The choice of column dimensions, such as length and diameter, depends on the separation scale and the desired resolution.

Chromatography System: A multimodal chromatography system includes various components to operate and control the separation process. This may include a pump for delivering the mobile phase, detectors for monitoring the eluting molecules, valves for sample injection, and a data acquisition system for collecting and analyzing chromatographic data.

Buffer Solutions: Buffer solutions are used to adjust the pH and ionic strength of the mobile phase to optimize the separation conditions. Buffers can be selected based on the specific interaction modes involved in the multimodal chromatography process, such as ion exchange or affinity interactions.

Analytical Techniques: Analytical techniques, such as UV-Vis spectroscopy, refractive index detection, fluorescence detection, or mass spectrometry, are employed to monitor the separation process and detect the eluting molecules. These techniques provide information about the purity, concentration, and identity of the separated components.

The specific combination and design of these components in multimodal chromatography can vary depending on the specific application and separation requirements. By integrating multiple interaction modes into the stationary phase, multimodal chromatography offers enhanced selectivity and versatility in separating and purifying target molecules.

Standard Operating Procedure of Multimodal Chromatography

Developing a specific Standard Operating Procedure (SOP) for multimodal chromatography will depend on the specific system and

HPLC Basics

method being used, as well as the requirements of the separation process. However, here is a general outline of the steps that can be included in an SOP for multimodal chromatography:

Column Preparation:

- ✓ Verify the integrity and cleanliness of the chromatography column.
- ✓ Equilibrate the column with an appropriate mobile phase to ensure the stationary phase is ready for sample loading.

Sample Preparation:

- ✓ Prepare the sample by properly diluting or concentrating it as needed.
- ✓ Filter the sample using a suitable filter to remove any particulate matter or impurities.

Mobile Phase Preparation:

- ✓ Prepare the mobile phase according to the specified composition and pH.
- ✓ Ensure the mobile phase is properly degassed to minimize the formation of air bubbles in the column.

System Setup:

- ✓ Ensure the chromatography system is properly calibrated and functional.
- ✓ Connect the column to the chromatography system and prime the system with the mobile phase.

Method Initialization:

- ✓ Enter the appropriate method parameters into the chromatography system software.

HPLC Basics

- ✓ Set the desired flow rate, gradient program, and detection settings based on the separation requirements.

Sample Loading:

- ✓ Inject the prepared sample onto the column using an autosampler or manual injection.
- ✓ Monitor the chromatogram to ensure proper sample loading and system stability.

Elution:

- ✓ Initiate the elution process by applying the predetermined gradient or isocratic conditions.
- ✓ Monitor the separation process using appropriate detection techniques and record the chromatographic data.

Washing and Regeneration:

- ✓ After the separation is complete, wash the column with suitable wash solutions to remove any residual sample or contaminants.
- ✓ Regenerate the column using recommended regeneration protocols to restore the stationary phase's performance and stability.

System Shutdown:

- ✓ Flush the column with an appropriate storage or equilibration solution to ensure its stability during storage.
- ✓ Properly clean and maintain the chromatography system and column according to the manufacturer's instructions.

Data Analysis and Documentation:

- ✓ Analyze the obtained chromatographic data using appropriate software tools.

✓ Document the results, including peak retention times, peak areas, and purity assessments.

It's important to note that this is a general outline, and the specific steps and parameters will vary based on the multimodal chromatography method being used. It is recommended to consult the manufacturer's guidelines, scientific literature, and experienced chromatographers for a comprehensive and customized SOP tailored to the specific multimodal chromatography system and application.

Limitations of Multimodal Chromatography

Multimodal chromatography has several advantages in terms of enhanced selectivity and improved purification efficiency. However, like any analytical technique, it also has certain limitations that should be considered. Some of the limitations of multimodal chromatography include:

Ligand Compatibility: The selection and compatibility of ligands used in multimodal chromatography can be critical. It is essential to ensure that the ligands used do not interfere with the stability, activity, or structure of the target molecule. Compatibility issues can arise when using harsh elution conditions or when the ligands interact with specific functional groups of the target molecule, leading to reduced recovery or altered conformation.

Ligand Leakage: Depending on the immobilization method and stationary phase design, there is a possibility of ligand leaching or detachment from the support material during the chromatographic process. Ligand leakage can result in decreased column performance, loss of selectivity, and increased batch-to-batch variability. Proper column preparation and storage conditions can help mitigate ligand leakage.

Limited Commercial Availability: Compared to traditional chromatographic methods, such as ion exchange or size exclusion chromatography, the availability of multimodal stationary phases and ligands may be relatively limited. The range of commercially available multimodal chromatography resins might be narrower, limiting the options for method development and optimization.

Matrix Effects: Multimodal chromatography can be susceptible to matrix effects, especially when dealing with complex samples or crude extracts. The presence of impurities, high salt concentrations, or other components in the sample matrix can affect the selectivity and performance of the multimodal chromatography system, leading to reduced resolution or compromised separation efficiency.

Method Development Challenges: Developing an optimized multimodal chromatography method can be complex and time-consuming. Finding the right combination of ligands, mobile phase composition, and gradient conditions to achieve the desired selectivity and resolution can require extensive experimentation and optimization. Method development may also involve evaluating different ligand densities, ligand ratios, and column dimensions to maximize separation performance.

Limited Scalability: Scaling up multimodal chromatography processes from laboratory-scale to large-scale production can pose challenges. Maintaining consistent performance and reproducibility across different column sizes can be difficult due to variations in mass transfer, pressure limitations, and other factors. Special considerations are needed to ensure scalability while preserving the selectivity and efficiency achieved at smaller scales.

Cost Considerations: Multimodal chromatography resins and ligands can be relatively expensive compared to traditional chromatographic media. The higher cost may limit the feasibility of using multimodal chromatography in certain applications, especially for large-scale purification processes.

It is important to assess and address these limitations when considering the application of multimodal chromatography in a specific context. Proper method development, optimization, and validation, as well as understanding the sample matrix and ligand compatibility, can help mitigate these limitations and maximize the benefits of multimodal chromatography.

www.ingramcontent.com/pod-product-compliance
Lightning Source LLC
Chambersburg PA
CBHW072232170526
45158CB00002BA/861